Diana Roberts

Mediterranean Diet

The 21-Day Quick & Easy Guide of
Low Carb Mediterranean Diet Meal Plan
and Recipes for Beginners to
Lose Weight Fast and for Optimum Health

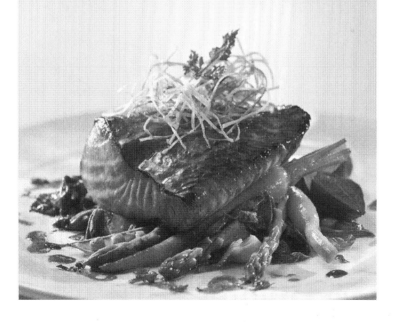

Copyright and Disclaimer

Copyright 2014 by Diana H. Roberts - All rights reserved.

Book Description

Have you been curious as to how to start the Mediterranean Diet, but don't have a clue as to where to start? With this quick start guide, you are sure to get off on the right foot from the beginning. Through these pages, you will learn what the Mediterranean Diet actually is, the foods you will need to focus on and the exercises that you can incorporate into your daily life in order to make your success at the Mediterranean Diet a reality.

Table of Contents

Introduction

Practically every day a new diet pops up in the world we live in. Companies are developing products to help us lose weight fast and special foods are being created just so that we can shed a few of those unwanted pounds. In this ever changing world, it becomes increasingly more difficult to find a diet plan that is both healthy and will help us to look our best.

It is time to throw out the get thin quick methods and return to something that has been proven successful time and time again. There is a reason that the people of the Mediterranean are some of the healthiest in the world; their diet. This diet is rich in things that are wholesome and healthy and switching to this diet can be simple and delicious.

Plus, you will not need to purchase a strange pill or contraption to help you succeed with this diet. Everything lies in the food that you eat, which are probably things that you already eat on a daily basis, just not in the right quantities.

As you take the journey into the Mediterranean Diet through this book, you will be able to learn exactly why it is beneficial and what makes it the best diet for many who are looking to be healthy and live longer. By the end of this book, you will have all the tools that you need to get started with your very own Mediterranean Diet and will easily be able to plan the meals that you choose to correspond with this lifestyle.

Chapter 1 – What is the Mediterranean Diet?

Even though the Mediterranean Diet became popular during the 90's, it wasn't officially recognized until the fall of 2010. This diet is inspired by Mediterranean cuisine from countries such as Greece, Spain, and Southern Italy.

This diet is low in saturated fat, but high in mono-saturated fat and dietary fiber, which helps people to lose weight, maintain a healthy weight and helps to reduce certain ailments, such as high blood pressure and cholesterol.

Saturated fat, even though it occurs naturally in foods, can raise cholesterol levels and increase the risk of heart disease and stroke. Research shows that limiting your saturated fat to less than 7% of your daily calories is the best way to eliminate these issues.

Saturated fat can be replaced by mono-saturated fats, which work to lower bad cholesterol in the blood. These fats are high in Vitamin E, which boosts the immune system because it acts like an antioxidant. This fat should still make up less than 25% to 35% of your total daily calories.

Dietary fibers help to improve the blood sugar and lower the blood pressure and bad cholesterol in the body. It also acts as a natural laxative to help rid the body of toxins and waste. It is recommended that women who are under the age of 50 consume 25 grams daily, while men consume 38 grams. Women over the age of 50 should reduce this amount to 21 grams and men should reduce theirs to 30.

With the Mediterranean diet, you will be focusing on dairy, grains with little or no saturated and Trans fat, nuts, seafood, and a number of spices. These items are all important when looking to maintain the Mediterranean diet and will help you to lose weight and to avoid many chronic health problems and diseases.

For dairy products, make sure that you stick to low-fat or fat-free options. It is a good idea to choose yogurt or cheese when planning your meals and consume 1 to 3 servings each. You can also use soy products as a replacement for traditional dairy products; however, it is recommended that you take a calcium and vitamin D supplement if you choose to go this route.

The most important portion of your Mediterranean diet should be whole grains, which will be about 4 to 6 servings each day. Not only are they high in fiber, but they will help keep you full for longer periods of time and can help you lose weight this way.

Another important component of the Mediterranean diet is nuts. They help protect against heart disease and stroke because they contain unsaturated fatty acids in omega-3. It is recommended that you choose one or two servings a day and avoid options that are salted or sweetened so that you can avoid calories and sugar.

Fruits and vegetables are also highly recommended and you should consume 4 to 8 servings each day. Although fresh items are preferred, fruits that are canned in light syrup or their own juices can be used as a replacement in some cases.

With the Mediterranean diet, red meat will be limited and it will be replaced with fish and shellfish that are high in omega-3. You should aim to have two or three servings of omega-3 rich fish per week. Poultry is also allowed, but you should only consume 1 to 3 servings each week. You will need to make sure that the poultry you choose is prepared without the skin. Red meats should be lean and limited to around 12 to 16 ounces per month.

Exercise is also important when adapting to this lifestyle. Walking is very popular, but gardening and other exercise methods are also recommended. You should get around two and a half hours each week when it comes to exercising, as a minimum.

By choosing the Mediterranean diet, you have the potential to remain healthy for many years. This is truly a lifestyle that you will need to adopt in order to keep your heart healthy. There are ways to make the plan more affordable, such as choosing frozen vegetables and buying nuts in bulk. However, it is best if you can stick with fresh fruits and vegetables. This diet has helped to create a lifestyle for the people in the Mediterranean that has led to some of the best longevity in the world.

Chapter 2 – Getting Started the Right Way

When you are starting out with the Mediterranean diet, the first thing that you need to do is to study the Mediterranean diet food. This will help you know the quantities of food that you should be consuming for each food group. For example, you will want to eat less meat and more fruits and vegetables. Below is an example that has been provided by the Mayo Clinic:

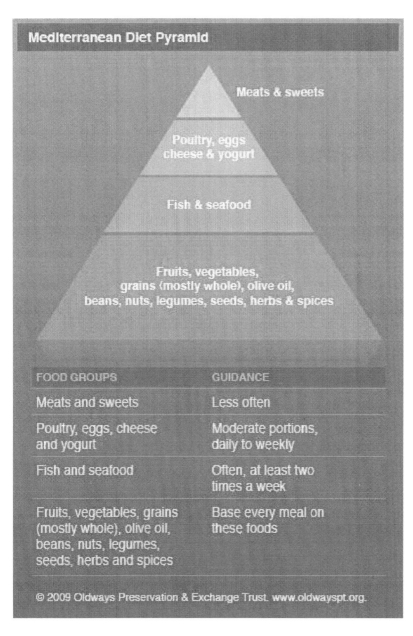

Mediterranean Diet Pyramid

Meats & sweets

Poultry, eggs
cheese & yogurt

Fish & seafood

Fruits, vegetables,
grains (mostly whole), olive oil,
beans, nuts, legumes, seeds, herbs & spices

FOOD GROUPS	GUIDANCE
Meats and sweets	Less often
Poultry, eggs, cheese and yogurt	Moderate portions, daily to weekly
Fish and seafood	Often, at least two times a week
Fruits, vegetables, grains (mostly whole), olive oil, beans, nuts, legumes, seeds, herbs and spices	Base every meal on these foods

Spend some time familiarizing yourself with the various items that are suggested throughout this diet. Make sure you learn about the different types of food that is commonly consumed in the Mediterranean and learn about how they benefit your body.

It is also a good idea to start out by talking to a dietitian so that you understand the correct amounts of vitamins and nutrients that you will need to take in addition to the diet that you will be starting. Below are a number of tips that can help you get started the right way.

- Begin by making a simple trade of butter for olive oil. This is a great substitute when you are sautéing vegetables. You can even drizzle it on salads or use it has a dip for bread if you mix it with fresh herbs. This will help you to lose cholesterol, but gain some of the heart healthy monounsaturated fats that are important to this diet.

- Next, you should start eliminating some of your red meat meals. Make a gradual transition by eating fish or seafood twice a week and by reducing the portions of the meat that you serve. You should also begin incorporating a vegetarian meal each week as well.

- Begin adding more vegetables to your meals. They are the main focus of the Mediterranean diet and you will need to begin the process of consuming them at lunch and dinner. You should aim to fill half of your plate with vegetables during this time. Start by focusing on vegetables that you already enjoy and begin introducing new options slowly. One tip is to try out a seasonal vegetable each week and prepare vegetables in a variety of different manners. Vegetables are great in salads and they are great when you grill, roast or sauté them. You can also add vegetables to pizzas, pasta dishes, soups and stews.

- Next, you will want to begin switching out your regular pasta for whole-grain options instead. Make sure that you check the ingredient list on the options at the grocery store and make sure that the first ingredient listed is whole. Whole grains provide vitamins, minerals, and fiber that are important for digestive help and there is a large variety of them that you can choose from.

- Finally, when you are ready to have a dessert, begin switching out cookies, cakes and ice cream for fresh fruit instead. You can still enjoy traditional sweets on special occasions, but for everyday sweet needs, make sure that you stick with healthy options.

The idea is to make daily changes gradually so that you can use yourself into this lifestyle over an extended period of time. It is best to make the change every week, so that you are ready to devote yourself to the diet after 21 days.

Chapter 3 – Shopping Guide

For a quick start guide, here are the top food items that you should add to your shopping list when beginning the Mediterranean diet.

Fish and Poultry

- Chicken

- Turkey

- Oysters

- Shrimp

- Salmon

- Squid

- Mackerel

- Mussels

- Tuna

- Lobster

- Tilapia

- Salmon

- Flounder

Healthy Fats
- Olive Oil

- Canola Oil

Vegetables
- Artichokes

- Eggplant

- Celery

- Broccoli

- Onions

- Peas

- Peppers

- Sweet potatoes

- Lettuce

- Mushrooms

- Celery

- Tomatoes

- Apples

- Cherries

- Dates

- Peaches

- Grapefruit

- Melons

- Strawberries

Dairy

- Low fat – fat free milk

- Low fat – fat free yogurt

- Low fat – fat free cheese

Grains

- Wheat

- Oats

- Couscous

- Rice

- Barley

- Bulgur

Beverages

- Red Wine (1 glass per day is permitted)

- Water

- (Avoid soft drinks and fruit juices)

Nuts

- Unsalted nuts

- Walnuts

- Pecans

Herbs and Spice

Instead of using salt and pepper for seasoning, the Mediterranean diet relies on certain spices and herbs to make food taste great.

- Anise

- Basil

- Bay

- Capers

- Cardamom

- Cinnamon

- Chervil

- Garlic

- Onion

- Cumin

- Saffron

- Sage

- Thyme

- Rosemary

- Sage

Chapter 4 – 21 Meals to Get You Started

One of the best things about the Mediterranean diet is that it is very versatile. For example, you can easily substitute foods that have been added to recipes depending on your particular palette. Simply make sure that the food that you are using to replace the original has the same calorie content of the food that you are replacing it with. Below, you will find 21 meals to get you started with the Mediterranean diet today.

Drinks

Calorie free drinks are allowed throughout the course of the diet. You can choose from water, diet iced tea, diet soda and flavored seltzer.

You should not exceed 3 cups of caffeinated coffee or 4 cups of caffeinated tea each day. In fact, the less you drink the better. However, you do not have to stick with decaffeinated coffee or tea. Do keep in mind, that there are 16 calories in each teaspoon of sugar and 21 calories in a small prepackaged container cream. To reduce some of these calories, switch to 1% milk that has about 6 calories per tablespoon and limit sugar to about 2 teaspoons each day.

Breakfast

1. Pancakes

Combine the following in a bowl: 1 ½ cups low-fat yogurt, an egg, 1 cup pancake mix (whole wheat or buckwheat) and ¾ cup fat free milk. Recipe will make 5 servings or 20 small pancakes. You can easily save the remaining servings for another meal by placing them in the freezer. To go with your pancakes, serve with 1 tablespoon of light maple syrup and garnish with a cup of fresh strawberries. For your drink, have 1 cup fat free milk.

2. Yogurt Granola Parfait

Layer 6 ounces of light, fruit flavored yogurt with 1 cup raspberries and 2 tablespoons granola. You will make three layers, so divided the ingredients in threes to make your layers.

3. Omelet with Salmon and Asparagus

Sauté 2 tablespoons of onion until translucent and add in two steamed asparagus spears, a minced clove of garlic, and a quarter teaspoon lemon juice for two minutes. In a separate bowl, mix a teaspoon of low-fat milk, two eggs, 1/2 tablespoons parsley and seasonings, such as salt, pepper, dill, and chives to taste. Add eggs to vegetable mixture and allow it to set. Add salmon and reduce heat. Cook for two or three minutes and fold in half. Continue cooking for one more additional minute.

4. Toast with Cheese, Fruit and Nuts

What you need: 1 slice of whole grain toast, ¾ oz. low calorie cheese, ½ pear and ½ tsp walnuts. Toast bread and top with other ingredients.

5. Granola with Fruit and Nuts

Mix ½ cup low fat granola with ½ cup low fat or fat free milk. Top with a quarter of a banana, a quarter of a medium apple and 1 tsp chopped walnuts.

6. Oatmeal with Fruit and Nuts

Mix ½ cup oats with 1 cup low fat or fat free milk. Microwave on high for 2 minutes and mix in 1 tsp almonds and sunflower seeds. Top with a quarter of a mango and half an apple.

7. Creamy and Crunch Yogurt

Top 6 ounces of light yogurt, any flavor, with 1 cup high fiber cereal (100 calories worth) and 3 tablespoons of chopped walnuts.

Lunch

1. Chickpea Salad

Mix together: ½ 15 ounce can of chickpeas (rinse in colander for a couple of minutes in order to remove sodium), 2 tsp extra virgin olive oil, ¼ cup white onion – chopped, ¼ cup green pepper – chopped, 1 tablespoon black olives – sliced, ¼ tsp black pepper and 1 ½ tablespoons white vinegar. Serve over 2 cups of romaine lettuce.

2. Vegetable Pot Pie

Serve 10 grape tomatoes with 1 Amy's or Swanson's Chicken or Vegetable Pot Pie that has been prepared according to the directions on the package.

3. Vegetarian Pita Sandwich – Greek Cucumber Yogurt Sauce

Mix ½ cup plain light yogurt and ½ finely chopped cucumber, ½ minced garlic clove and a bit of salt and pepper. Spread half of this mixture on 6 ½ inch whole wheat pita and fill with 1 cup string beans and 5 halved grape tomatoes. Serve with 1 cup cherries.

4. Pizza and Salad

Pair 1 slice of thin crust pizza with vegetable toppings with a minimum 2 cup green salad. Top with 2 tablespoons of dressing (any variety) and have a scoop of ice cream for dessert.

5. Lentil Soup

Boil 5 cups of water, 2 tablespoons of salt, 2 tablespoons olive oil, a dash of saffron, ½ cup chopped white onion and 1 cup red lentils for about 15 minutes. Add 1 tsp cumin and cook for another 5 minutes. Serve with a small salad and fruit.

6. Orange Salad

Place shredded lettuce on a plate and layer with thinly sliced oranges, onions and olives. Combine 2 tablespoons olive oil, 2 tsp lemon juice, a bit of salt and pepper for a dressing.

7. Fresh tomato Penne

Mix 8 tomatoes (seeded and chopped) with a cup of green onions, crumbled feta cheese, chopped parsley, chopped dill and a quarter cup of extra virgin olive oil. Boil 12 oz. penne pasta until it is tender but firm. Toss mixture together with drained pasta and season with salt and pepper.

Dinner

1. Chicken Kabobs

What you need: 4 ounces of raw chicken breast chunks, onion and green pepper chunks, grape tomatoes and ¼ cup fat free Italian dressing. Marinate chicken in dressing a minimum of 30 minutes. Place chicken, onion, green pepper and tomatoes on skewer and grill. Serve with a Pita that has been topped with 2 tablespoons hummus.

2. Tomato and Mozzarella Sandwich

Sprinkle 1/3 cup of reduced-fat shredded mozzarella cheese onto halves of a 6 inch French baguette roll and toast in toaster oven. After the bread has been toasted, sprinkle dried basil and oregano on halves and top with tomato slices.

3. Spaghetti with Tomato Sauce

Sauté a clove of crushed garlic and a pinch of red pepper flakes in olive oil until garlic turns golden brown. Add 7 oz. crushed tomatoes and cook for 10 minutes. Add in 4 oz. cooked spaghetti and sprinkle with a tablespoon grated Parmesan.

4. Salmon with orange and lemon

Combine 2 tsp each of orange, lemon juice, and olive oil with 1 tsp soy sauce. Add in your salmon and allow to marinate for about 15 minutes. Cook in broiler for about 10 to 12 minutes and use any remaining juices to spoon over salmon.

5. Grilled Swordfish

Brush 4 oz. swordfish with a tablespoon of olive oil and salt and pepper. Broil for 7 to 8 minutes before pouring on a mixture of: 2 tablespoons olive oil, 1 tablespoon lemon juice, ¼ tsp crushed garlic, splash of soy sauce and a pinch of oregano; broil for one additional minute.

6. Broiled Chicken with Garlic and Live

Rub chicken with a combination of 2 minced garlic cloves, ½ tsp salt and 1 ½ tbsp. of lime juice and allow to marinate for 1 hour. Broil chicken in oven, turning every 5 minutes, until chicken is no longer pink.

7. Basil Shrimp Summer Salad

Marinate 3 oz. shrimp in a basil marinade for a minimum of 30 minutes. Marinade consists of: ¼ cup white vinegar, 1 tsp olive oil, 1 tbsp. lemon juice, and 1/8 cup chopped fresh basil (1 tsp dried basil). Grill shrimp and top with 2 cups of romaine lettuce. Serve with a cup of blueberries.

Snacks

Crackers and Dip

1 cracker with 2 tablespoons humus and pair with a fresh plum

Chickpea spread

This is for two servings so you can save one serving for the next day. Mash half a can of chickpeas in a bowl with a fork slightly. Mix in the following: 2 teaspoons olive oil, a clove of minced garlic, a tablespoon of lemon juice, and a quarter teaspoon of salt and a quarter teaspoon of ground cumin (optional). Mix well and if you are looking for a smoother spread, you can put the ingredients into a food processor. For dipping, you can bring a cup of broccoli or peppers along with your spread.

Chapter 5 – Fun Recipes to try

You will find some very fun recipes that you can try to incorporate the Mediterranean Diet into your own life. However, here are a few that can be fun and delicious. Be sure to try some of them out when you are beginning your journey.

Poached Pears

Looking for that perfect dessert to pair with your fantastic new lifestyle? This simple approach will pair with any meal nicely.

Ingredients
1 cup orange juice
¼ cup apple juice
1 tsp, each ground cinnamon and nutmeg
4 whole pears
½ cup raspberries
2 tablespoons of orange zest

Preparation
1. Combine juices and spices in small bowl; mix evenly by stirring
2. Peel pears – leave stem, but remove the core
3. Add pears and juice mixture to shallow pan
4. Simmer, over medium heat for 30 minutes (turn pears frequently – don't boil)

5. Serve immediately. Garnish with raspberries and orange zest

Mediterranean Salad

If you are looking for a fantastic recipe to replace the brown bag special that you are used to consuming at lunch, this is it. It's simple and delicious and can easily be made for a large gathering or a simple weekday lunch.

Note: One of the best things about this salad is that you can make it as small or as large as you like. This recipe has been designed for 2, but it is simple to increase the size of it to make it fitting for the entire family.

Ingredients
¾ sliced and seeded cucumbers
¼ cup and 2 tablespoons feta cheese – crumbled
¼ cup pitted and sliced black olives
¾ cups Roma tomatoes – diced
1 tablespoon and 1 tsp diced sundried tomatoes – packed in oil (drain and reserve oil)
1/8 sliced red onion

Preparation
1. In a large bowl, toss all ingredients together with a small portion of the sun-dried tomato oil that you reserved. Chill until you are ready to serve.

Seafood Couscous Paella

With only 409 calories per serving and 7 grams of fat, this saffron-infused couscous makes a fantastic dinner. It is filling and can easily be modified to fit any budget or taste preference.

Ingredients:
2 teaspoons olive oil (extra-virgin)
1 chopped medium onion
1 minced clove of garlic
½ tsp dried thyme
½ tsp fennel seed
¼ tsp salt
¼ tsp ground pepper
A pinch of crumbled saffron threads
1 cup diced tomatoes (no salt added, with juice)
¼ cup vegetable broth
4 ounces bay scallops (tour muscle removed)
4 ounces small shrimp (peeled and deveined)
½ cup whole-wheat couscous

Preparation

1. Over medium heat, heat oil in large saucepan
2. Add onion – stir constantly while you cook for 3 minutes
3. Add and cook for 20 seconds:
    a. Garlic
    b. Thyme
    c. Fennel seed
    d. Salt
    e. Pepper
    f. Saffron
4. Stir in tomatoes and broth
5. Bring to a simmer. Cover and reduce heat for 2 minutes
6. Return heat to medium and stir in scallops

7. Stir constantly for 2 minutes
8. Repeat process with shrimp
9. Stir in couscous and remove from heat
10. Cover and allow it to sit for 5 minutes before fluffing and serving.

Chapter 6 – Exercising with the Mediterranean Diet

Exercise is an important part of the Mediterranean diet. People in this section of the world are known for their healthy lifestyle as well as the healthy way that they exercise regularly.

Some of the best ways to gain this exercise is through normal, everyday activities, such as walking, gardening, and other physical activities. However, there are also some specific exercises that you can try to help strengthen your muscles and get in shape.

It is suggested that you combine some strength training exercises along with your weekly exercise program. Below are some examples of some of the exercises that you can rely on when you are working out while living the Mediterranean diet lifestyle.

The Ball Squeeze

This exercise has been designed to work out your inner thighs and all you need is an exercise ball and some floor space. Start by lying on your back and placing your hands behind your ears. Next, you will raise your legs into the air and slightly bend your knees. Place the exercise ball between your legs, in between your feet and your knees. Engage your abdominal muscles and squeeze the ball slightly with your thighs for 10 seconds. Relax for five seconds and then repeat the process for a total of five sets.

Knee Swimmer

For this exercise, you will begin on your hands and knees. Keep your knees about hip width apart and your hands should be shoulder width apart. Your fingers will be facing forward. While keeping your back flat and your head down, lift out your left leg, straight behind you and reach your right arm in front of you. Don't forget to keep your back straight and your stomach muscles engaged. After you have completed the left side switch to the right side and complete 10 full sets.

Triceps Press

When you begin this exercise, start with your feet fit hip width apart. You also need to have a single dumbbell that you hold in both hands. Raise your arms over your head, making sure that your palms face the ceiling and your thumbs are intertwined. Next, you should slowly bend your elbows and lower the weight behind your head. You will need to keep your elbows as steady as you can. Finally, you should raise the weight slowly back into the starting position. For this exercise, you will complete two sets and 12 repetitions.

Floor Oblique

When attempting to work your core muscles, this exercise is a fantastic option. Start by lying on your left side on the floor and keep your back straight. Your legs will be stretched out behind you. Prop your right leg on top of your left leg and move your legs to a 45° angle in front of your body and bend your knees slightly. Your left arm will be placed in front of your body for balance and you will place your bent right arm on your ear. Now you should lift your torso into a crunch towards your hips. With this exercise, you will be able to work out your side abdominal muscles. After you return to your starting position complete 10 repetitions and change sides to complete two sets per side.

Downward Dog

Start this exercise on your hands and knees with your hands shoulder width apart and your knees hip width apart. Next, you will curl your toes up so that your body resembles an upside down letter V. Make sure your head is between your arms and look at your feet, making sure to keep your weight distributed between your feet and your hands. You can increase the stretch by pushing your heels towards the floor and pushing your butt further into the air. You should try to keep your back as flat as possible and your head relaxed while you hold this pose for 30 seconds.

Spinal Twist

This exercise will help elongate your back and outer thigh muscles. Start by sitting on the floor and stretching your legs out in front of you. Your arms will be down by your side. Bring your left foot over your right leg bending your left knee. Keep your back straight and rotate your torso to the right so that your right arm crosses in front of the rest of your body. Rest your right elbow against your left thigh, above the knee and put your left arm behind you for support. You can rotate your upper body further to make this stretch deeper. Hold this pose for 30 seconds and then switch to the other side to repeat.

Pigeon

With this exercise, you will start out as you did with the Downward Dog. Your body will resemble an upside down V. However, with this exercise you will bring your right leg underneath you as you keep your leg bent. Your knee should be at the center of your chest and your left leg will be stretched out behind you. Now, you will sit up while keeping your upper body straight and holding your arms along your side for balance. For this stretch, you can make the stretch deeper if you push your hips towards the ground, which will lower and stretch your entire upper body out in front of you. Allow your chest to touch your right leg upper thigh and you can touch the floor with your forehead, as long as your arms are stretched out in front of you. Hold this pose for 30 seconds before repeating for the other side.

There are a number of exercises that you can incorporate with the Mediterranean diet. The trick is to simply get exercise as much as possible while you're on this diet. It is a major part of the lifestyle and has many benefits for the people who participate in it.

Other than the general benefits that you normally see with exercise, combining the Mediterranean diet with exercise has shown many other benefits as well. For example, studies have shown that those combining a healthy exercise program and the Mediterranean diet have a lower risk of developing mental issues, such as Alzheimer's disease. In fact, those who stick with the Mediterranean diet and follow a physically active lifestyle are 60% to 70% less likely to develop Alzheimer's disease.

Conclusion

The Mediterranean Diet is a fantastic way of life that has kept people healthy for centuries. It is so successful because there are no gimmicks that are involved and you can start it today without subscribing to a meal plan or buying a particular product.

If you start today, you will quickly learn the benefits for yourself and will be able to begin living the healthy lifestyle that is enjoyed by people all across the Mediterranean region. Now is the time to begin transforming yourself into the person that you want to be and you now have all the tools to do so.

Whether you are ready to start small or dive into a full lifestyle makeover, try out some of the foods from the shopping guide to get started. There are plenty of recipes available, other than those listed in this book, for you to enjoy today.

With some dedication and a fun cooking strategy, this diet can be the one that finally works and you will be able to see yourself transform before your very eyes. Don't wait a moment longer before you begin living the healthy life today. Start a Mediterranean Diet and see just how healthy you can be.

As with any diet, it is a good idea to discuss your plans with your doctor so that you can be certain that you are receiving all the proper nutrients and vitamins that you need to remain healthy. Since everyone is made differently, there may be different items that you need in relation to certain medications that you are taking or certain medical issues that you may have. Make sure that your doctor is aware of changes that you are making to your lifestyle so that you can remain healthy for the years to come.

Check Out Other Related Book

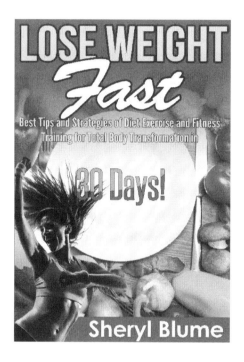

This book contains proven steps and strategies to transform your physical and mental approach to weight loss.

Millions of people all around the world are dieting as we speak, they may have started today, yesterday, last week – for some really dedicated individuals maybe even last month. They all have one thing in common though; the unfortunate truth is they are likely to fail.

There is one very simple reason for this, while they are addressing what goes into their mouths on a daily basis their not addressing the area that really controls the outcomes we gain in life....the mind.

Within this book we're going to give you the exact tools you need to do just that, were also going to show you how to apply them to your life instantly so that over the next 30 days the entire direction of your future can be altered for the better.

Made in the USA
Monee, IL
12 October 2023